My Mediterranean Soup

*50 Delicious Soups & Other Mouth-Watering
Recipes for Your Mediterranean Daily Meals*

Alex Brawn

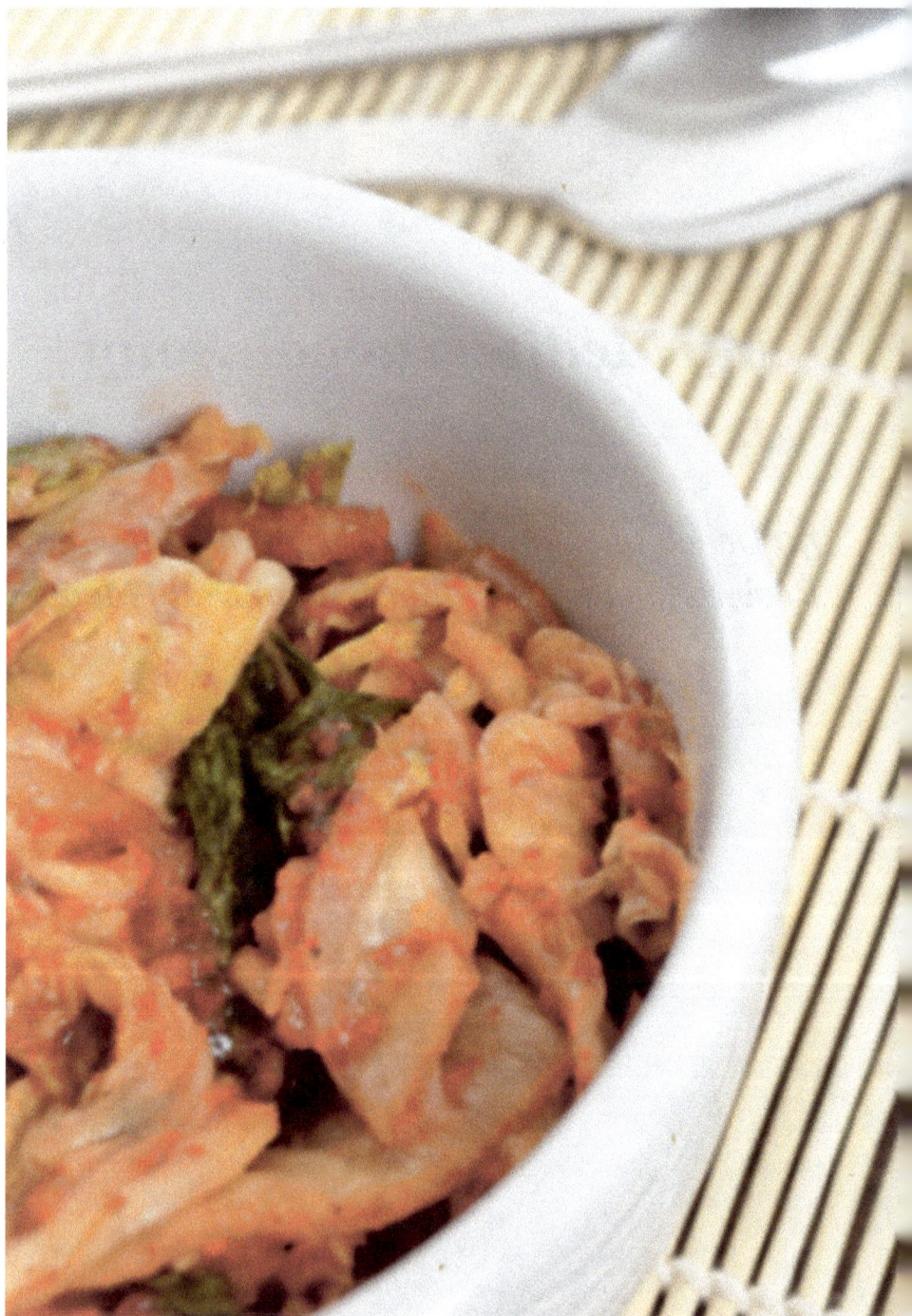

Table of Contents

Roast carrot and fennel soup

Ingredients

- ½ teaspoon of dried yeast
- 1kg of carrots
- 250g of strong bread flour
- 1 onion
- 1 teaspoon of fennel seeds
- 1 teaspoon of sugar
- Olive oil
- 2 cloves of garlic
- 1.6 liters of organic vegetable stock
- 2 bulbs of fennel
- 100ml of single cream

Directions

- Preheat your oven to 375°F.
- Place carrots, onion, and fennel in a roasting dish, toss with 2 tablespoons of oil.
- Roast for 20 minutes, add the unpeeled garlic cloves.

- Stir vigorously and return to the oven for further 20 minutes, or until the vegetables are soft.
- Discard garlic cloves.
- Put the roasted vegetables in a large pan with the vegetable stock and bring to the boil.
- Then, Simmer gently for 15 minutes, liquidize with a stick blender, until smooth.
- Toast the fennel seeds in a dry frying pan briefly until fragrant.
- Crush roughly, pour into a bowl with the flour and sea salt.
- Dissolve the yeast and sugar in in hot water.
- Add to the flour mixture with the olive oil and hot water and mix until dough foams, knead.
- Divide the dough into 8 and roughly roll each one into a thin oval.
- Stack them up, separating them with baking paper.
- Heat a griddle pan until it's smoking hot, add the flatbreads.

- Cook for briefly on each side, until charred and puffed up.
- Serve and enjoy.

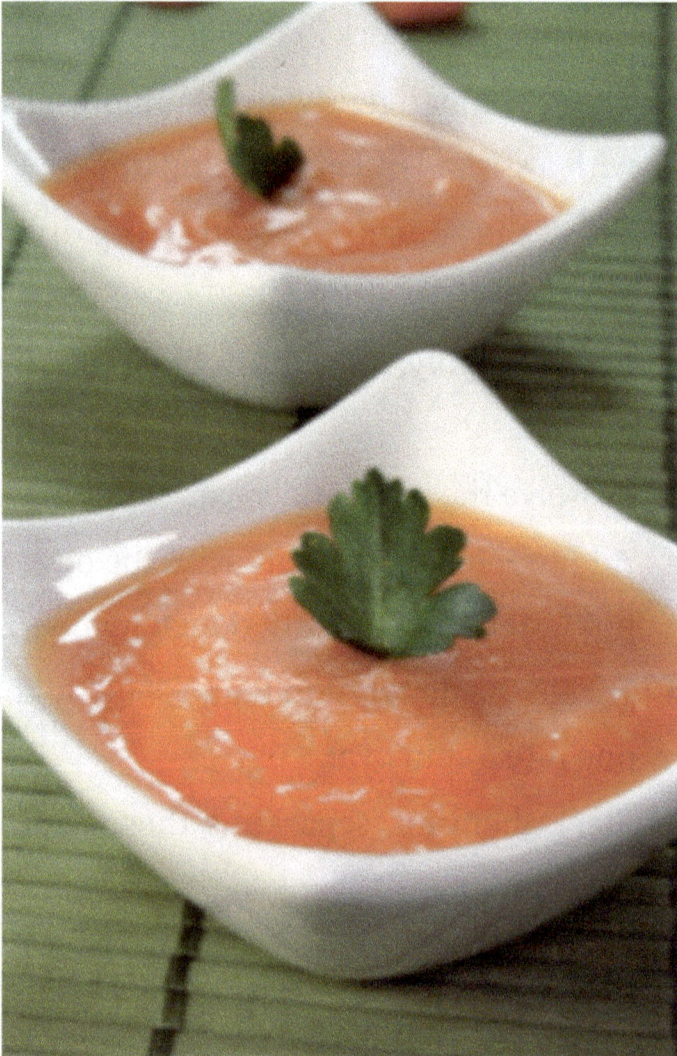

Chicken and vegetables soup

Ingredients

- 1 chicken carcass and bones
- 2 large onions
- 2 sticks of celery
- 1 leek
- Olive oil
- 2 sticks of celery
- 1 bunch of fresh flat-leaf parsley
- 5 black peppercorns
- 4 carrots
- 1 bunch of fresh flat-leaf parsley
- 2 courgette
- 200g of cooked chicken
- 100g of orzo
- 50g of frozen peas

Directions

- Place in a large saucepan quartered onions, with chicken carcass, carrots, celery, peppercorns, and parsley.

- Cover with cold water, season with a little sea salt.
- Bring to the boil over a medium heat, skimming any froth off the surface.
- Lower heat and simmer slowly for 3 hours when covered.
- Strain the broth, let cool.
- Add a splash of oil to a separate large saucepan and place over a medium heat.
- Add onion, leek, celery, carrots, courgette, and parsley. Sauté for 5 minutes.
- Stir in the orzo and stock, bring to a boil.
- Lower the heat and simmer until the veggies are cooked.
- Stir in the peas and chicken until heated through.
- Season to taste.
- Serve and enjoy.

Store cupboard lentil soup

Ingredients

- 1 organic vegetable stock cube
- 2 red onions
- ½ teaspoon dried thyme
- 200g of dried lentils
- Olive oil
- 2 carrots
- 1 x 410 g tin of cannellini beans
- 3 sticks celery
- ½ a dried chili
- 2 cloves garlic
- 6 rashers of smoked streaky bacon
- A few sprigs fresh flat-leaf parsley

Directions

- Heat olive oil over a medium heat
- Add the bacon and fry slowly until crispy, then crumble in the dried chili, dried thyme, carrot, celery, onion, and garlic.
- Cook gently for about 15 minutes covered until all the vegetables are soft.

- Add the lentils with a liter of water.
- Bring to the boil and simmer until the lentils are soft.
- Drain, then place in the cannellini beans.
- Bring back to the boil and simmer for another 10 minutes.
- Season with sea salt and black pepper.
- Add into bowls and drizzle with extra virgin olive oil and the chopped parsley.
- Serve and enjoy.

Ribollita

Ingredients

- 310g of cavelo Nero
- 1 bay leaf
- 2 large handfuls of good-quality stale bread
- 1 ripe tomato
- 1 pinch of dried red chili
- 1 small potato
- Extra virgin olive oil
- 1 x 400g tin of plum tomatoes
- 2 small red onions
- 2 carrots
- 3 cloves of garlic
- 3 sticks of celery
- Olive oil
- 1 pinch of ground fennel seeds

Directions

- Place beans in a pan with bay leaf, tomatoes, and potatoes cook until the beans are tender. Drain and discard the bay leaf, tomato and potato. Reserve some bean water.

- Heat a saucepan with a splash of olive oil.
- Add the vegetables to the pan together with the ground fennel seeds and chili.
- Sweat very slowly on a low heat with the lid just ajar for 20 minutes until soft.
- Add the tomatoes and bring to a gentle simmer briefly.
- Add the cooked and drained beans with a little of the reserved water, bring back to the boil.
- Moisten and stir the bread.
- Continue cooking for about 30 minutes.
- Season with sea salt and black pepper.
- Stir in extra virgin olive oil.
- Serve and enjoy.

Corn chowder soup

Ingredients

- 1 medium potato, peeled and cut into little cubes
- 3 spring onions
- 1 medium onion
- Olive oil
- ½ teaspoon of dried thyme
- ¼ cup of fresh chives, chopped, or parsley
- 1 stalk celery
- 175g of frozen corn
- 1 tablespoon of plain flour
- 840ml of semi-skimmed milk

Directions

- Heat the olive oil in a medium saucepan over a medium heat.
- Add the celery, onion, and thyme.
- Stir until vegetables start to brown.
- Sprinkle the flour over the veggies and stir briefly.

- Pour in the milk, then add the potato let boil, stirring the whole time so the soup, until the potatoes are tender in 10 minutes.
- When the potatoes are tender, stir in the corn together with the spring onion and celery leaves.
- Bring the soup back to the boil.
- Serve and enjoy with crusty brown bread.

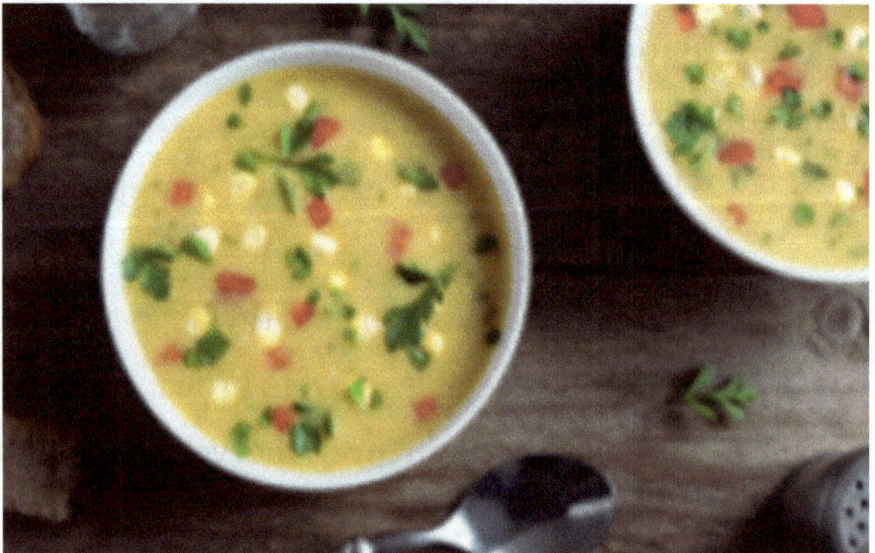

Roasted cauliflower and coconut soup

Ingredients

- 600g of cauliflower
- 1 x 400g tin of reduced-fat coconut milk
- 1 heaped teaspoon of ras el hanout
- 4 cloves of garlic
- 1 heaped teaspoon of ground cinnamon
- 3 tablespoons of chili oil
- Olive oil
- 1 handful of unsweetened coconut flakes
- 2 onions
- 600ml of vegetable stock

Directions

- Preheat your oven to 350°F.
- Place the onions, cauliflower in a roasting tray with the unpeeled garlic cloves and sprinkle with the cinnamon and ras el hanout.
- Season, then drizzle with olive oil.
- Toss, and place into the oven for 30 minutes, or until cooked through.

- Scatter the coconut flakes on to a small tray, place briefly into the oven to toast.
- When the vegetables are ready, remove the garlic cloves and scrape all the vegetables into a large saucepan.
- Squeeze the garlic out of its skins and add to the mixture.
- Pour in the coconut milk with stock, bring to the boil.
- Lower the heat, let simmer for 5 minutes.
- Blend the soup until creamy and smooth, adjust with water if too thick.
- Taste and adjust the seasoning.
- Serve and enjoy topped with the toasted coconut flakes and a drizzle of chili oil.

Chicken noodle soup

Ingredients

- 1 pinch of saffron
- Dry sherry
- Sweet ginger vinegar
- 200g of small carrots
- 100g of baby leeks
- 1 handful of fresh parsley stalks
- 300g of mixed fine pasta shapes
- 2 cloves of garlic
- 2-3 fresh bay leaves
- 200g of small onions
- 1 celery heart
- 5cm of piece of ginger
- 1 x 1.4kg of whole free-range chicken

Directions

- Place celery, carrots, garlic, and onions into a very large saucepan with the chicken, bay leaves, and parsley stalks.
- Season with sea salt and black pepper, then add enough water to cover the chicken.

- Bring to the boil, lower the heat down, let simmer for 1 hour.
- Empty the pan except for stock, then shred the chicken.
- Bring the stock back to the boil and add a good splash of sherry with the saffron and a splash of ginger vinegar.
- Add the pasta and continue to boil until the pasta is al dente.
- Return the chicken and vegetables to the pan and simmer over low heat until warmed through.
- Serve and enjoy.

Clear Asian noodle soup with prawns

Ingredients

- 1 carrot
- 100g of runner beans
- 2 large free-range eggs
- 250g of brown rice noodles
- 200g of cooked peeled king prawns
- 3cm piece of ginger
- 2 fresh hot Thai chilies
- 2 liters of organic chicken stock
- 2 tablespoons of sesame seeds
- 2 tablespoons of low-salt soy sauce
- 6 radishes
- 4 spring onions
- 2 cloves of garlic
- 2-star anise
- 6 cloves

Directions

- Start by cooking the eggs in boiling water for 5 minutes.

- Let cool under cold running water, peel and keep aside.
- Cook the noodles according to the package Directions, drain, leave in a dish of cold water.
- Add ginger and chili to a large pot together with the stock, unpeeled garlic cloves, soy sauce, star anise, and cloves.
- Bring to a simmer, put off the heat, let infuse for 20 minutes.
- Cook runner beans with carrot in a pan of boiling water for 2 minutes.
- Drain, then plunge into cold water.
- Strain the stock into a clean pot, return to a medium heat, then add sliced prawns.
- Cook until just heated through.
- Toast the onions and radishes with the sesame seeds in a dry frying pan.
- Drain the rice noodles and divide between 4 bowls.
- Sit the beans, carrot, and prawns on top.

- Place over the broth and top with the radishes, spring onions, half an egg, and toasted sesame seeds.
- Serve and enjoy.

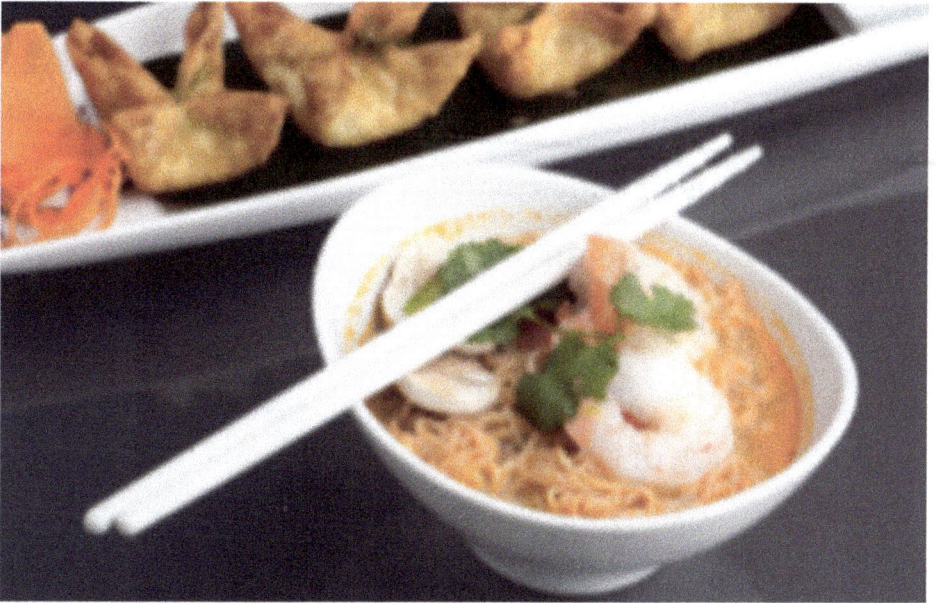

Sweet potato, coconut, and cardamom soup

Ingredients

- 1 pinch of dried chili flakes
- 1 teaspoon of coriander seeds
- 3 green cardamom pods
- 2 jarred roasted peppers
- 800ml of organic vegetable
- 1 onion
- 100g of baby spinach
- 1 x 400ml tin of low-fat coconut milk
- 4cm piece of ginger
- 4 large poppadum
- 600g of sweet potato
- 2 cloves of garlic
- 3 tablespoons of groundnut oil
- 1 lemon

Directions

- Crush the cardamom seeds in a mortar.
- Heat groundnut oil over a low heat, then add the onion with a small pinch of sea salt let cook

for 10 minutes in a large saucepan, stirring often.

- Stir in the sweet potato together with the ginger, garlic, and crushed cardamom seeds.
- Let cook for 2 minutes, then add the coconut milk.
- Allow it to simmer for 2 minutes, stir in the stock.
- Cover with a lid, and leave to simmer gently for 15 minutes.
- Liquidize the soup in a blender until smooth.
- Season with a pinch of salt and black pepper and a squeeze of lemon juice.
- Heat groundnut oil in a frying pan, add crushed coriander seeds and chili flakes.
- Let cook for 1 minute.
- In a dry pan, toast the coconut flakes.
- Add sliced peppers to the spices with the spinach.
- Continue cooking until the spinach has wilted down.
- Season and stir in the toasted coconut flakes.

- Place the soup into bowls
- Serve and enjoy topped with red pepper.

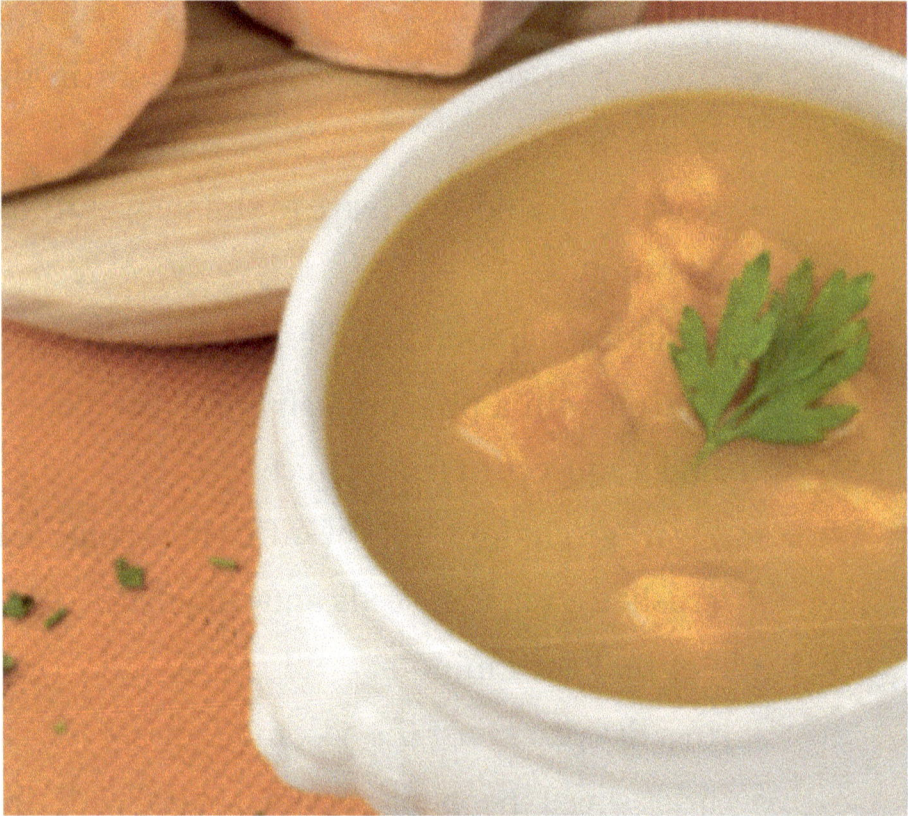

Beetroot and tomato borscht

Ingredients

- 2 celery stalks
- 1 clove of garlic
- 1.2 liters of organic beef stock
- 2 tablespoons of tomato purée
- A few sprigs of fresh dill
- 1 teaspoon of caster sugar
- 1 x 400g tin of plum tomatoes
- 2 large beetroot
- ½ of a small red cabbage
- 2 carrots
- 4 tablespoons of sour cream
- 1 red onion

Directions

- Begin by pouring tomatoes into a large pan, stir in the onion with carrots, celery, garlic, beef stock, beetroot, tomato purée, and sugar.
- Bring to the boil and simmer gently for 5 minutes.

- Add the shredded cabbage, let simmer for another 30 minutes or so.
- Blend the soup until smooth.
- Serve and enjoy hot with swirls of the sour cream, then sprinkled with chopped dill.

Pistou soup

Ingredients

- 6 sprigs of fresh basil
- 60g of Parmesan cheese
- 1 onion
- 1 x 400g tin of borlotti beans
- 8 cloves of garlic
- 3 leeks
- 7 tablespoons of extra virgin olive oil
- 1 x 400g tin of cannellini beans
- 3 potatoes
- 3 carrots
- 1 stick of celery
- 3 courgettes
- 2 sprigs of fresh flat-leaf parsley
- 2 fresh bay leaves
- 250g of baby green beans
- 1 x 400g tin of chopped tomatoes
- 70g of small macaroni

Directions

- Start by heating the olive oil over a medium heat.
- Sauté the onion with garlic and leek for 5 minutes.
- Add the potatoes, carrots, courgette, and celery, bay, green beans and chopped tomatoes.
- Drain and add the beans.
- Cover with water, then season, let simmer until the vegetables are tender.
- Then, add the pasta and simmer until cooked. Regulate water as needed.
- Place garlic, basil leaves, and sea salt in the mortar.
- Pound until puréed, then finely grate in the Parmesan.
- Muddle in the extra virgin olive oil to make a paste.
- Serve and enjoy.

Celeriac and quince soup

Ingredients

- 2 banana shallots
- 1 teaspoon of ground cumin
- 2 cloves of garlic
- olive oil
- A few sprigs of fresh dill
- 1 organic chicken stock cube
- 1 teaspoon of sugar
- 1 quince
- 1 small handful of walnuts
- 1 tablespoon of crème fraiche
- 1 pinch of ground cinnamon
- 1 large celeriac

Directions

- Place olive oil to a large pan, put over a medium-low heat.
- Add the celeriac, shallots, garlic, cumin, cinnamon, sugar, and quince, crumbling in the stock cube.

- Let cook gently for 25 minutes, stirring occasionally.
- Add in enough boiling water to cover the vegetables once all vegetables have softened.
- Uncover and let simmer for 25 minutes, or until the vegetables are cooked through.
- Blend to your preferred consistency.
- Roughly chop the walnuts and toast in a little butter.
- Then, top the soup with a swirl of crème fraiche, a little picked dill and a handful of chopped toasted walnuts.
- Serve and enjoy.

Red lentil, sweet potato, and coconut soup

Ingredients

- ½ a bunch of fresh coriander
- 1 liter of organic vegetable stock
- 750g of sweet potatoes
- 1 x 400g tin of light coconut milk
- 2 red onions
- 125g of red lentils
- ½ tablespoon of cumin seeds
- 1 teaspoon of ground coriander
- Olive oil
- 1 lemon
- 4 cloves of garlic
- 1 fresh red chili

Directions

- Preheat the oven to 350°F.
- Place sweet potatoes with onion wedges in a roasting tray in an even manner.
- Sprinkle over the cumin seeds with ground coriander and a pinch of sea salt and black pepper.

- Then, drizzle with oil, toss to coat.
- Place in the oven for 45 minutes, or until golden.
- Place a large saucepan over a medium-low heat and pour in a lug of oil.
- Sauté the garlic together with the chili and coriander stalks briefly, until lightly golden.
- Add the red lentils to the pan.
- Stir to coat, then pour in the hot stock with coconut milk.
- Raise the heat, let boil, then simmer.
- Cook the lentils for 20 minutes.
- Remove from the oven when veggies are ready, spoon into the pan.
- Add most of the coriander leaves, then blend the soup until creamy with some little texture.
- Taste and adjust the seasoning with lemon juice.
- Serve and enjoy with coriander leaves.

Spiced parsnip and lentil soup with chili oil

Ingredients

- 3 tablespoons of groundnut oil
- 1 small smoked ham hock
- A few sprigs of fresh mint
- 1 onion
- 1 garlic clove
- Fat-free Greek yoghurt
- 3cm piece of ginger
- 400g of parsnips
- Olive oil
- 250g of red lentils
- 2 red chilies
- 2 tablespoons of Rogan paste
- 1.6 liters of organic vegetable stock

Directions

- Soak the ham hock in cold water overnight.
- Drain and place it in a saucepan.
- Cover with cold water, bring it to the boil.
- Lower the heat, let simmer for 2 hours.

- Drain again, and set aside.
- Place the groundnut oil in a pan over a very low heat.
- Add sliced garlic and chilies to the pan, warm for 5 minutes.
- Heat olive oil in a large pan, then add the onion.
- let cook gently for 5 minutes, stirring frequently.
- Add the parsnips together with the rogan paste and ginger, let cook for 5 minutes.
- Add the lentils, stock, and the ham hock, bring to the boil.
- Simmer for about 30 minutes, until the lentils soften.
- Remove and discard the ham bone and liquidize the soup until smooth.
- Return any lean ham to the saucepan and reheat.
- Shred the mint leaves and serve scattered on top of the soup with a dollop of yoghurt.
- Serve and enjoy.

Caldo Verde

Ingredients

- Paprika
- 1 large onion
- Extra virgin olive oil
- 2 cloves of garlic
- 300g of kale
- 150g of chorizo
- 700g of potatoes

Directions

- Start by heating 4 tablespoons of oil in over medium heat.
- Fry the onion with garlic for 5 minutes, or till soft.
- Stir in the potatoes, then season with sea salt, let cook for 5 minutes.
- Add water, then simmer for 20 minutes.
- Then, mash the potatoes into the liquid to produce a smooth purée.
- Add the kale, let simmer for 5 minutes.

- Heat 1 tablespoon of oil in a frying pan over medium heat.
- Fry the chorizo slices, sprinkling with paprika in the pan for 4 minutes.
- Add the chorizo to the soup.
- Place the soup into bowls and season with freshly ground black pepper.
- Serve and enjoy with slices of corn bread.

Baked potato soup

Ingredients

- Sour cream
- 3 large baking potatoes
- 1 Parmesan rind
- 40g of butter
- 1.5 liters of organic chicken
- 1 small bunch of fresh chives
- 1 onion

Directions

- Preheat the oven to 360°F.
- Prick cleaned potatoes with a fork and wrap in foil.
- Place on a rack in the middle of the oven, let cook for about 1 hour 15 minutes.
- Remove, when cool enough, cut into quarters. Let cool completely.
- Melt butter over a medium-low heat, add and cook diced onion for 10 minutes.
- Add the potato with Parmesan rind to the pan.
- Season, and cook for 5 minutes.

- Add the stock, bring to the boil.
- Lower the heat, let simmer for 30 minutes.
- Remove, purée the soup until smooth without the rind.
- Return to the pan.
- Taste, and adjust the seasoning.
- Serve and enjoy with a dollop of sour cream, snipped chives and a pinch of black pepper.

Caprese soup

Ingredients

- 1½ tablespoons red wine vinegar
- 50g of basil leaves
- 1 bulb of garlic
- 4 slices of sourdough bread
- 1kg of mixed tomatoes
- Extra virgin olive oil
- 2 x 125g of balls of buffalo mozzarella
- 4 sun-dried tomatoes in oil
- 1 tablespoon of soft brown sugar

Ingredients

- Preheat the oven ready to 400°F.
- Place cut garlic in a large roasting tray with the tomatoes.
- Drizzle with 1 tablespoon of olive oil.
- Let roast in the oven for 25 minutes, or until the tomatoes have burst.
- Let cool totally.

- Squeeze and roasted garlic into a blender with the roasted tomatoes, sugar, basil, sun-dried tomatoes, vinegar, and 3 tablespoons of oil.
- Blend until smooth, then transfer to a jug.
- Heat a griddle pan and chargrill the sourdough on both sides.
- Serve and enjoy with half a torn mozzarella ball in the center topping with basil leaves and cracked black pepper.

Goulash soup

Ingredients

- 1 tablespoon of tomato purée
- 250g of onions
- 2 cloves of garlic
- ½ tablespoon of caraway seeds
- 200g of potatoes
- 1 green pepper
- 2 tomatoes
- Sour cream
- A few sprigs of fresh marjoram
- Extra virgin olive oil
- 500g of beef shin
- Red wine vinegar
- 1 tablespoon paprika
- 1½ liters of organic beef stock

Directions

- Place a splash of extra olive oil in a large pan.
- Sauté the onions with garlic and pepper until softened.

- Add the beef and continue to cook until the meat is browned and the vegetables are cooked.
- Then, stir in the paprika, let cook for 2 minutes.
- Add the beef stock.
- Bring to the boil until reduced by half.
- Add the marjoram together with the tomatoes, the tomato purée, caraway seeds, a splash of vinegar, season well.
- Add enough stock to cover, let simmer until the meat and vegetables are tender, in 2 hours.
- Add diced potatoes, with the remaining stock.
- Let simmer until the potatoes are cooked.
- Serve and enjoy with a dollop of sour cream.

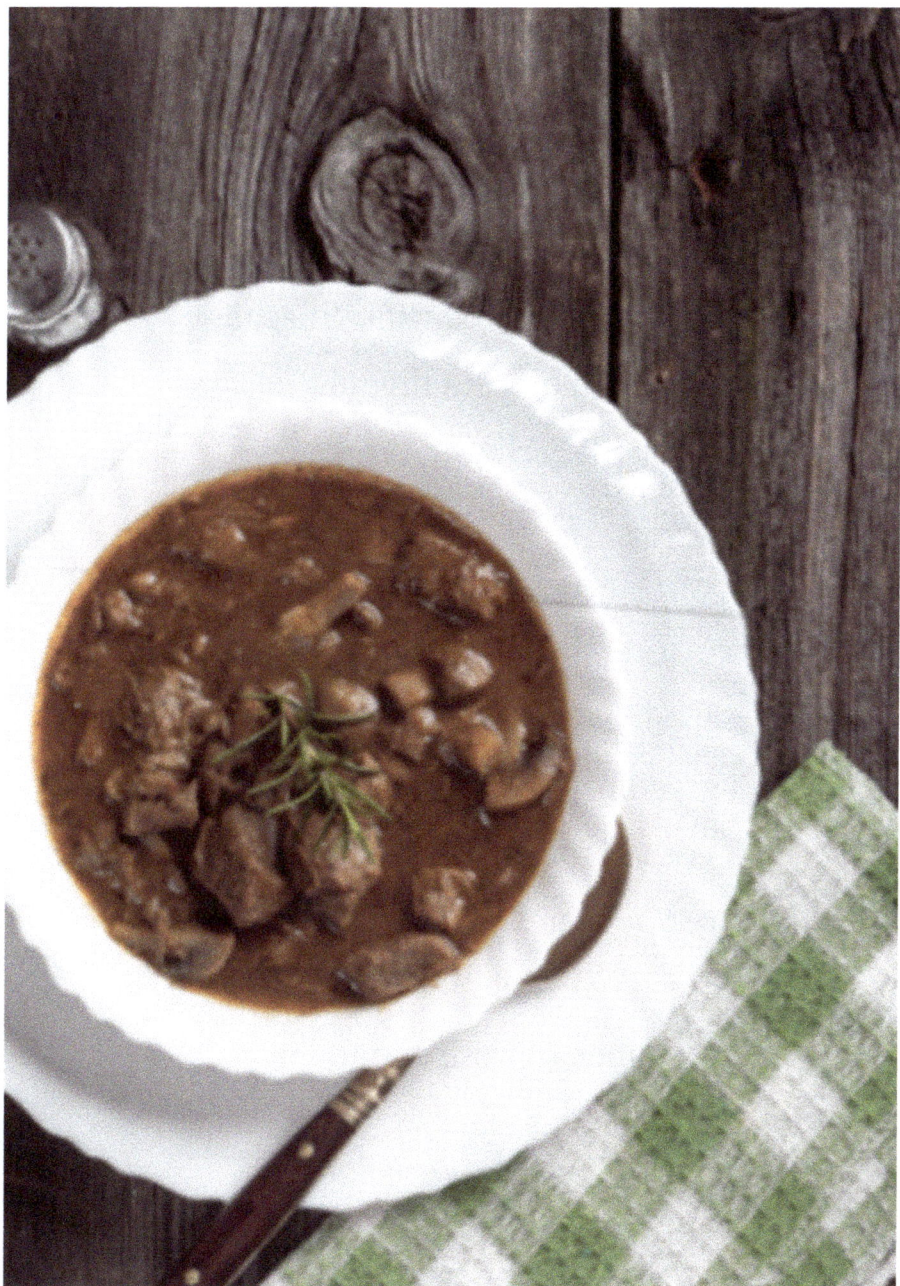

Costa Rican black bean soup

Ingredients

- 4 large free-range eggs
- 3 red onions
- 1 tablespoon of red wine vinegar
- ½ a bunch of fresh thyme
- 2 cloves of garlic
- 2 sticks of celery
- Extra virgin olive oil
- 2 x 400g tins of black beans
- 2 fresh bay leaves
- 1 green pepper
- 4 corn of tortillas
- 1 red pepper
- 2 fresh red chilies
- ½ a bunch of fresh coriander
- Olive oil

Directions

- Drizzle olive oil in a large saucepan over a medium-low heat.

- Add 2/3 of chopped onion, garlic, celery, coriander stalks, and peppers and thyme leaves to the pan.
- Add ½ of chili, gently sauté the veggies for 15 minutes.
- Place black beans with their liquid, bay leaves, and boiling water.
- Raise the heat and bring to the boil.
- Season well.
- Lower the heat, let simmer, for 30 minutes covered, or until creamy.
- Then, crack the eggs directly into the soup over reduced the heat.
- Leave the eggs to poach in the soup for 5 minutes.
- Add chopped coriander with remaining chopped onion, red wine vinegar, and a few tablespoons of extra virgin olive oil. Mix well.
- Serve and enjoy with black bean soup.

Mulligatawny soup

Ingredients

- 1 x 400g tin of chopped tomatoes
- 1 large onion
- 2 cloves of garlic
- 500g leftover of free-range turkey
- 750ml of hot organic chicken
- 1 carrot
- 300g of butternut squash
- 300g of basmati rice
- 1 thumb-sized piece of ginger
- 1 tablespoon of tomato purée
- 1 tablespoon of olive oil
- a few sprigs of fresh coriander
- 1 dried red chili
- 1 tablespoon of curry paste

Directions

- Firstly, heat olive oil in a large saucepan over a medium heat.
- Add the onion together with the garlic, carrot, ginger, and dried chili.

- Cover, and cook, stirring occasionally, until all the vegetables are soft and lightly golden.
- Then, add the butternut squash with tomato purée and curry paste, shred in the turkey, and stir to coat.
- Add the chopped tomatoes.
- Season with sea salt and black pepper.
- Pour in the hot stock and bring to the boil.
- Lower heat and let simmer for 15 minutes.
- Add the basmati rice and simmer for a further 10 minutes.
- Serve and enjoy garnished with coriander leaves.

Turkey and coconut milk soup

Ingredients

- 100g of oyster mushrooms
- 3 Thai shallots
- 200g of cooked, skinless turkey
- 2 bird's-eye chilies
- 1 thumb-sized piece of galangal or ginger
- 3 kaffir lime leaves
- 2 tablespoons of fish sauce
- 3 coriander roots
- A few sprigs of fresh coriander
- 2 lemongrass stalks
- 500 ml organic turkey
- 1 x 400ml tin of light coconut milk
- 1 teaspoon of palm
- 1/2 lime

Directions

- Add the stock with the coconut milk to a large saucepan.
- Bring to the boil, then turn down the heat.

- Add the sugar together with the chilies, lime leaves, lemongrass, shallots, galangal or ginger, and coriander roots.
- Season and simmer gently for 5 minutes.
- Add torn mushroom and shredded turkey to the pan.
- Lower the heat to low.
- Simmer for 3 minutes, and add the fish sauce and lime juice.
- Serve and enjoy hot with some coriander leaves.

Roasted carrot and fennel soup

Ingredients

- ½ teaspoon of dried yeast
- 1 teaspoon of sugar
- 1 teaspoon of fennel seeds
- 1kg of carrots
- 100ml of single cream
- 250g of strong bread flour
- 1 onion
- 2 bulbs of fennel
- Olive oil
- 2 cloves of garlic
- 1.6 liters of organic vegetable stock

Directions

- Preheat the oven to 375°F.
- Place sliced carrots, onion, and fennel in a roasting dish, and toss bit of oil.
- Let roast for 20 minutes, add the unpeeled garlic cloves.
- Stir, return to the oven for 20 more minutes, or until the vegetables are browned.

- Remove, discard the papery skins from the garlic cloves.
- Put the roasted veggies in a large pan with the vegetable stock, bring to the boil.
- Then, simmer for 15 minutes, then liquidize with a stick blender, until completely smooth.
- Toast the fennel seeds in a dry frying pan for 30 seconds.
- Crush roughly with mortar, then pour into a bowl with the flour and sea salt.
- Dissolve the yeast and sugar in hot water.
- Add to the flour mixture with the oil and hot water, mix until dough foams. Knead for 5 minutes.
- Place the dough into an oiled bowl, cover with oiled Clingfilm and set aside to rise.
- Divide the dough into 8, roll each one into a thin oval.
- Stack up, separating them with baking paper.
- Heat a griddle pan until very hot.
- Add the flatbreads let cook briefly on each side, until charred.

- Serve and enjoy with a swirl of cream, a scattering of herby fennel tops.

Steaming ramen

Ingredients

- 8 chicken wings
- 1 handful of pork bones
- 200ml of low-salt soy sauce
- 2 sheets of wakame seaweed
- 750g of pork belly
- 2 thumb-sized pieces of ginger

Sesame oil

- 1 thumb-sized piece of ginger
- 1 splash of mirin
- 1 heaped tablespoon of miso paste
- 400g of baby spinach
- 500g of dried soba
- 8 tablespoons of kimchee
- 8 small handfuls of beansprouts
- 4-star anise
- 8 spring onions
- 7 garlic
- 2 fresh red chilies
- Chili oil

- 4 large free-range eggs

Directions

- Boil the eggs for 5 minutes.
- Pour the soy sauce, mirin, and star anise, with water into a small pan.
- Boil ginger and garlic, remove from the heat, then, pour the mixture into a sandwich bag with the eggs.
- Place in refrigerator for 6 hours, then drain.
- Preheat the oven to 400°F.
- Place chicken wings together with the pork bones into a large casserole pan.
- Bash, add the unpeeled ginger and garlic.
- Toss with a good drizzle of sesame oil.
- Place the pork skin on a baking tray, bake for around 40 minutes.
- Cover pork belly and miso with water, bring to the boil.
- Simmer over low heat for 3 hours, or until the pork belly is tender, skimming occasionally.
- Lift the pork belly onto a tray and put aside.

- Sieve the broth and pour back into the pan. Return to the heat and reduce the liquid down.
- Place a large colander over the pan and steam the spinach until wilted.
- In another separate pan, cook the noodles according to packet Directions, drain.
- Divide between 8 large warm bowls with the beansprouts and spinach.
- Taste the broth and adjust the seasoning.
- Tear over the seaweed and divide up the kimchee.
- Serve and enjoy drizzle with chili oil.

Apple and celeriac soup

Ingredients

- 200ml of crème fraiche
- 4 tablespoon of olive oil
- 2 onions
- 2 liters of vegetable stock
- A few sage leaves
- 1 celery stalk
- Toasted hazelnuts
- 1 celeriac
- 4 apples
- A few sprigs of thyme

Directions

- Heat half of the olive oil in a large pan.
- Add sliced onions, celery, let cook over a medium heat for 10 minutes until soft.
- Add Chopped celeriac, apples, and thyme leaves to the pan, let cook for 2 to 3 minutes.
- Add the stock and season.
- Let simmer over a low heat for 30 minutes.
- Remove, and blend until smooth.

- Then, stir in half the crème fraiche.
- Heat the remaining olive oil in a pan, fry the sage leaves until crispy.
- Spoon the soup into bowls and top with the remaining crème fraiche.
- Serve and enjoy with a drizzle of extra virgin olive oil, sprinkled with the crispy sage leaves and hazelnuts

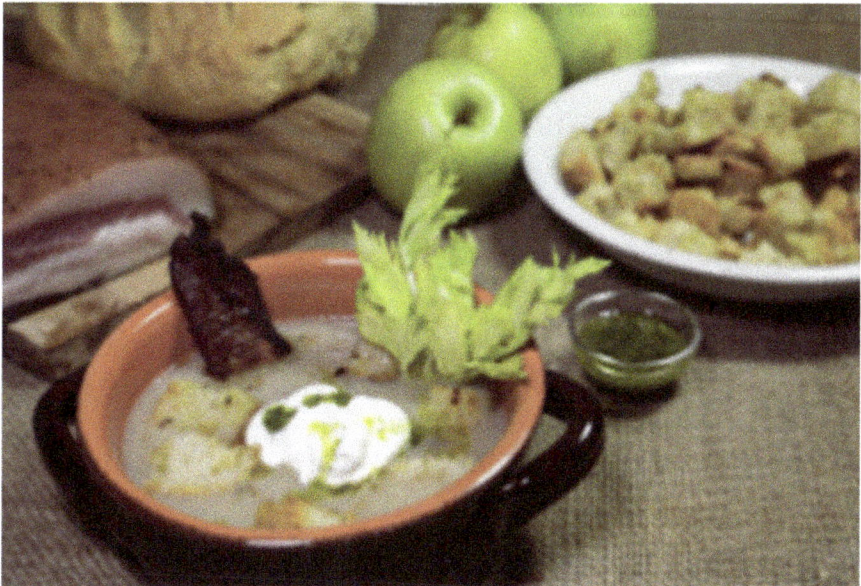

Roasted tomatoes and bread soup

Ingredients

- 2kg of ripe tomatoes
- ½ a bulb of garlic
- 2 red onions
- 1 pinch of dried oregano
- Olive oil
- 1 liter of organic vegetable stock
- A few sprigs of fresh basil
- 1 x 280g of ciabatta loaf
- Red wine vinegar
- Extra virgin olive oil

Directions

- Preheat the oven to 400°F.
- Place cut tomatoes on a large roasting tray.
- Scatter garlic bulbs and wedges of onions into the tray.
- Sprinkle with oregano.
- Season with sea salt and black pepper.
- Drizzle with oil, then let roast for 1 hour, or until the tomatoes sticky.

- Pour in the stock, roughly chop and add the basil stalks with most of the leaves.
- Tear 1 half of ciabatta loaf into the soup.
- Bring to the boil, simmer for 10 minutes.
- Heat a griddle pan to high.
- Slice the remaining ciabatta and griddle until lightly charred on both sides.
- Add 1 splash of red wine vinegar to the soup.
- Blend until fairly smooth.
- Ladle into bowls, drizzle with extra virgin olive oil and scatter with the remaining basil leaves.
- Serve and enjoy with griddled ciabatta on the side.

Garden glut soup

Ingredients

- 1 organic vegetable stock cube
- 1 medium onion
- 100g of podded fresh peas
- A2 sticks of celery
- a few sprigs of fresh mint
- 1 medium leek
- 200g of baby spinach
- 2 cloves of garlic
- Olive oil
- 3 medium potatoes

Directions

- Combine chopped onion, celery, garlic, and leek in a small bowel.
- Place a large pot on a medium heat with 2 tablespoons of olive oil.
- When hot, add vegetables the in the small bowl, lower the heat and cook with the lid askew for 10 to 15 minutes, stirring occasionally.

- Place chopped potatoes, courgette in a bowl.
- Fill and boil the kettle.
- Add the potatoes, courgettes, once the vegetables are cooked, with a tiny pinch of sea salt and black pepper.
- Crumble the stock cube into a measuring jug.
- Top up the boiling water and stir until dissolved.
- Pour the hot stock into the pot.
- Raise the heat to high and bring to the boil.
- Cook over low heat for 15 to 20 minutes or until the potato is cooked through.
- Add the peas with spinach and cook for 4 more minutes.
- Remove the pot to a heatproof surface, let rest.
- Blend until smooth.
- Ladle the soup into bowls and sprinkle over the mint.
- Serve and enjoy.

Asian noodles broth with fish

Ingredients

- 2 fresh red chilies
- 250g of fresh egg noodles
- 2 limes, juice
- Sea salt
- Low-salt soy sauce
- 220g can of water shell nuts
- Freshly ground black pepper
- Sesame oil
- Vegetable oil
- 2 cloves garlic
- 1 small bunch fresh coriander
- 1 thumb-sized piece of fresh ginger
- 100g of mange tout
- 1 liter of organic fish
- 500g of sole fillets

Directions

- Bring a pan of salted water to the boil.
- Place in and cook the noodles as instructed on the pack.

- Drain the noodles in a colander, toss in a little sesame oil.
- Divide the noodles between four scrving bowls.
- Heat a large frying pan over a medium heat.
- Add a splash of vegetable oil.
- Stir-fry the garlic together with the ginger, mange tout, water shell nuts, and half the chilies for 2 minutes.
- Add the hot stock and bring to the boil.
- Place in the sole pieces, cook for a minute.
- Season generously with soy sauce and black pepper.
- Serve and enjoy.

Brown Windsor soup with pearl barley

Ingredients

- 1 tablespoon of plain flour
- 1 large knob of unsalted butter
- Olive oil
- 2 liters of organic beef stock
- 1 fresh bay leaf
- 500g of diced stewing steak
- 1 tablespoon of Marmite
- 2 carrots
- 150g of pearl barley
- 1 splash of Worcestershire sauce
- 1 sprig of fresh rosemary
- 1 red onion
- 3 sticks of celery

Directions

- Melt the butter in a large pan over a medium heat.
- Add a splash of olive oil with the steak, and lightly brown the meat.

- Stir in the Marmite with the Worcestershire sauce.
- Raise the heat to high and keep stirring until all the liquid has evaporated.
- Add carrots together with the onions, bay leaf, rosemary sprig, and celery, cook over a low heat covered until soft.
- Stir in the flour, pour in the stock.
- Season well with sea salt and black pepper.
- Bring to the boil, lower the heat to let simmer.
- Add the pearl barley, let cook gently for 1 hour.
- Remove, then discard the rosemary sprig with bay leaf.
- Whisk the soup to thicken.
- Serve and enjoy with hunks of soda bread.

Chicken garden soup

Ingredients

- A few sprigs of fresh flat-leaf parsley
- 2 onions
- 200g of baby spinach
- 6 carrots
- 2 handfuls of seasonal greens
- 6 sticks of celery
- 1 lemon
- 1 large knob of unsalted butter
- 2 fresh bay leaves
- 4 shallots
- 4 whole peppercorns
- 2 cloves of garlic
- 1 free-range of roast chicken carcass
- Olive oil

Directions

- Put chopped onions, carrots, celery, bay leaves, peppercorns, chicken carcass, and a pinch of salt in a bowl.

- Fill the pan with cold water, then place on a high heat and bring to the boil.
- Lower the heat, let a simmer and cook for 1 hour, skimming off any scum.
- About 20 minutes before the stock is ready, crack on with the base of the soup.
- Place the butter with 1 tablespoon of oil in a separate large pan on a low heat.
- Add the garlic together with the shallots and parsley stalks, let cook for 10 minutes.
- Add the carrots with celery, cook for a further 5 minutes.
- When the stock is ready, remove the chicken carcass with any remaining pieces of meat and leave to one side. Throw the carcass.
- Strain the stock through a sieve into the veggie pan.
- Bring to the boil, then reduce heat, simmer for 20 minutes.
- Add the seasonal greens, cook for 10 minutes.
- Add the spinach in the last minute.

- Divide between bowls and top with any leftover shredded chicken.
- Serve and enjoy sprinkled with parsley leaves and black pepper.

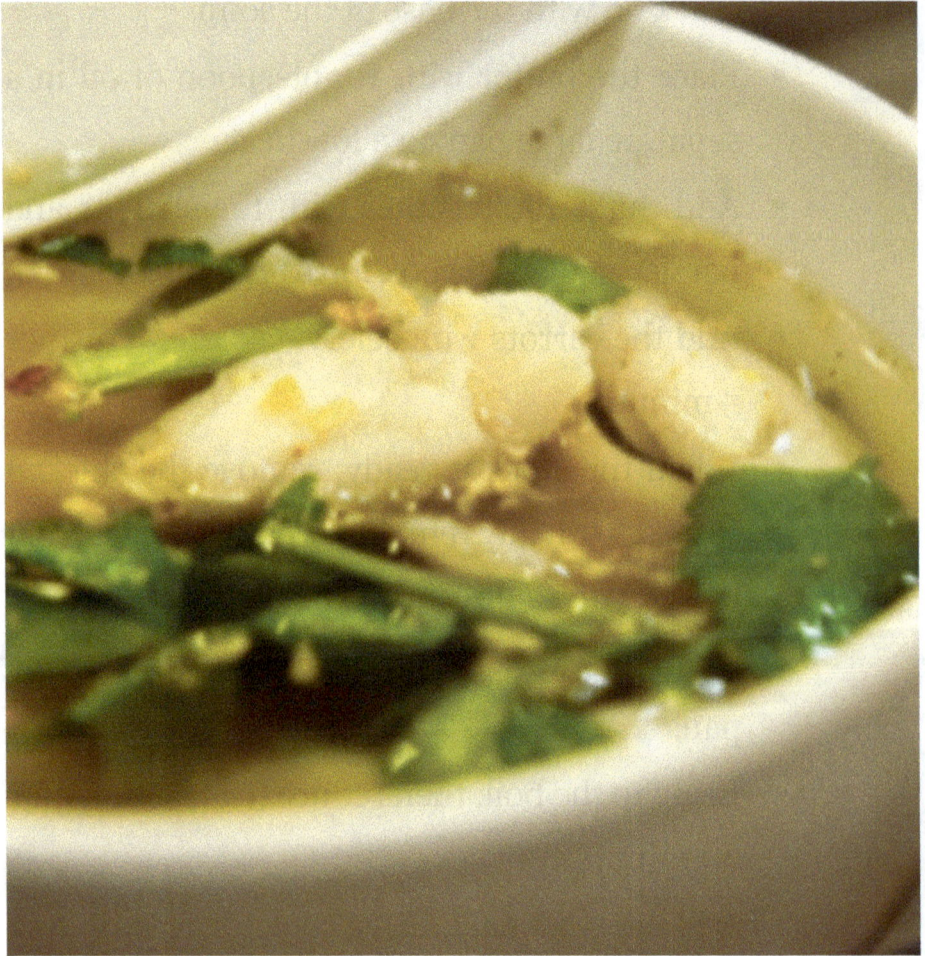

Chunky squash and chickpea soup

Ingredients

- 1 dried red chili
- Sea salt
- A few sprigs of fresh mint
- Olive oil
- 2 sticks celery
- 1 tablespoon of cumin seeds
- Harissa paste
- 2 lemons, zest
- 3 cloves garlic
- A few sprigs of fresh flat-leaf parsley
- 1 butternut squash
- 2 small red onions
- Extra virgin olive oil
- 1.5 liters of organic chicken
- 2 x 400g of tinned chickpeas
- 50g of almond flakes
- ½ tablespoon of fennel seeds
- ½ tablespoon of sesame seeds
- ½ tablespoon of poppy seeds

- Freshly ground black pepper

Directions

- Begin by preheating your oven ready to 400°F.
- Place the squash together with the cumin, and crumbled chili on to a baking tray.
- Drizzle with olive oil, mix together and place in the preheated oven.
- Roast for 45 minutes until the squash is cooked through.
- Heat a large saucepan once the squash is roasted, pour in a splash of oil.
- Add the celery together with the garlic, parsley stalks, and 2/3 of the onion, cook gently until softened, covered.
- Place in the roasted squash and let it sweat for a few minutes
- Pour in the stock. Bring to the boil.
- Let simmer for 15 minutes over low heat.
- Add the chickpeas and simmer for 15 minutes more.

- Toast the reserved squash seeds with the almond flakes, fennel, sesame, and poppy seeds in a little olive oil until all colored.
- Season, then blend briefly to thickens.
- Mix lemon zest together with the chopped parsley leaves, and mint leaves.
- Chop the remaining onion until it's really fine, add to zesty mixture, mix.
- Spoon half a teaspoon of harissa paste into each bowl.
- Divide the zesty herb mixture between the bowls and ladle over the soup.
- Stir each bowl with a spoon
- Serve and enjoy with the toasted seeds and almonds

Coconut millet bowl with berbere spiced squash and chickpeas

This is a plant based Mediterranean Sea diet that features shallots, spinach, millet grain, and coconut milk with vibrant flavors and spices.

Ingredients

- water
- 1 ½ lb. kabocha squash 3/4 slices
- 2 large shallots, sliced
- 1 cup of millet
- 1 teaspoon of grated fresh ginger
- 1 tablespoon of coconut oil
- ¼ cup of fresh mint leaves
- ¼ teaspoon of turmeric
- ¼ teaspoon salt
- ½ cup of fresh cilantro
- 15 oz. can chickpeas, drained
- 3 cups of fresh spinach
- ½ cup of coconut cream
- 2 tablespoons avocado oil
- ¼ cup of lime juice

- zest of one lime
- 1 teaspoon <u>honey</u>
- 2 tablespoons <u>Berbere spice</u>
- 1 cup of <u>coconut milk</u>
- ½ cup of cucumber chunks

Directions

- Set your oven to 400°F.
- Combine <u>berbere</u> , olive oil, and water in a bowl, hydrate for 10 minutes.
- Set aside some <u>coconut milk</u> .
- Boil the remaining <u>coconut milk</u> mixed with water, turmeric, and <u>salt</u> to a simmer.
- Add <u>coconut oil</u> with millet bring to a gentle boil, lower heat, let simmer for 15 minutes covered.
- Place prepared squash, shallots and chickpeas on <u>sheet pan</u> with <u>parchment</u> .
- Spread the <u>berbere</u> paste with a brush.
- Sprinkle with <u>salt</u> and place in oven for 30 minutes.

- Combine and blend the reserved coconut cream, <u>salt</u>, <u>honey</u>, cucumber, lime juice, and zest, and fresh ginger until smooth.
- Add the cilantro and mint, blend for few seconds.
- Assemble the bowls with the veggies on top of the warm millet.
- Then, add fresh spinach and drizzle with the sauce.
- Serve and enjoy.

Instant pot pinto bean stew

Ingredients

- 1 teaspoon of <u>chipotle powder</u>
- 2 teaspoons Molasses
- 1 tablespoon of olive oil
- 1 teaspoon of <u>salt</u>
- 1 large onion, chopped
- 4 cups of chopped poblano peppers
- 1 yam
- 4 cloves garlic coarsely chopped
- 14 oz. can of crushed tomatoes
- 3 cups of <u>veggie broth</u>
- 2 teaspoons of Ancho chili powder
- 1 cup of frozen corn
- 1 teaspoon of <u>cumin</u>
- 1 ½ cups of dry pinto beans
- 1 teaspoon of <u>coriander</u>

<u>Directions</u>

- Set instant pot to Sauté.
- Then, add olive oil with the onion, let sauté 5 minutes.

- Add garlic and poblanos continue to sauté for 2 minutes.
- Add the ancho chili powder together with the cumin, and coriander, stirring to coat.
- Add the yams together with soaked beans, molasses, chipotle, tomatoes, chicken stock, and salt .
- Set the Instant Pot to high pressure for 25 minutes.
- Manually release pressure valve.
- Stir in frozen corn and let warm through.
- Serve and enjoy.

Curried zucchini soup

Ingredients

- 2 teaspoons of <u>yellow curry powder</u>
- 2 tablespoons of <u>coconut oil</u>
- ¼ cup of cilantro- leaves
- 1 medium onion
- 2 cloves garlic
- 4 cups of chicken
- ¼ cup of mint leaves
- 1 tablespoon of ginger
- 1 jalapeño
- 1 ½ teaspoons of <u>sea salt</u>
- 2 pounds of zucchini or yellow squash

Directions

- In a heavy-bottomed pot sauté onion with garlic, ginger, and jalapeño in <u>coconut oil</u>, for 5 minutes over medium heat.
- Add the <u>salt</u> together with the zucchini and curry powder.
- Sauté briefly.
- Add 2 cups of the broth.

- Let simmer, covered and cook until the summer squash is tender.
- Add another 2 cups of cold broth to the <u>blender</u> with all the simmered ingredients.
- Blend, until smooth with a vented lid.
- Add fresh mint and cilantro, blend to incorporated.
- Serve and enjoy.

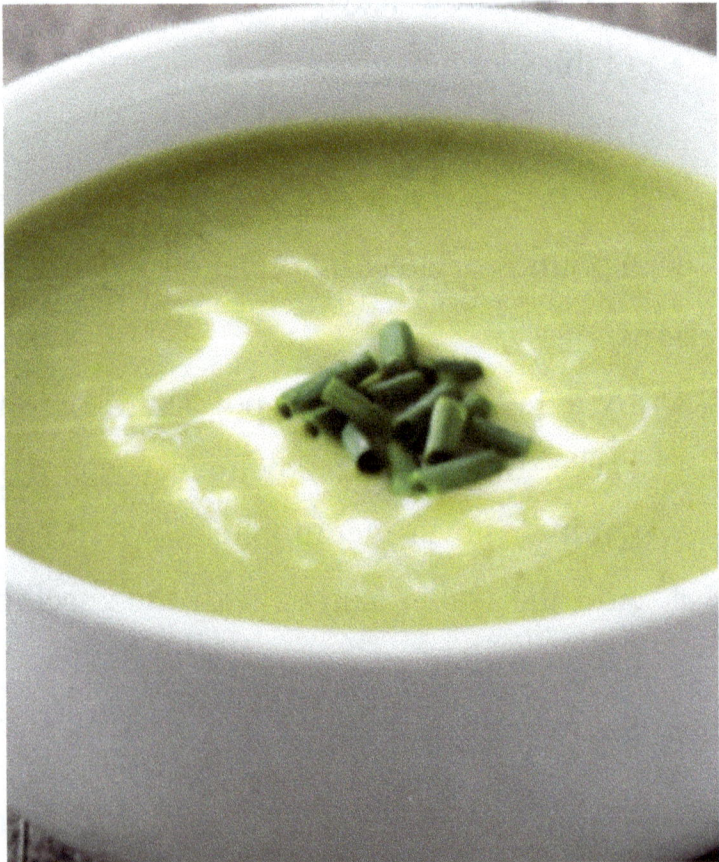

White bean chili with jackfruit

Ingredients

- 1 teaspoon of salt
- 1 tablespoon of coriander
- 1 tablespoon of cumin
- 2 tablespoons of olive oil
- 1 teaspoon of sugar
- 2 teaspoons of granulated garlic
- ½ teaspoon of pepper
- 1 onion, chopped
- 6 garlic cloves, rough chopped
- 2 teaspoons of dried oregano
- 1 poblano pepper, chopped
- 2 x 14-ounce cans of white beans
- ½ teaspoon of ground chipotle powder
- 16 ounces of canned jackfruit
- 3 cups of veggie broth
- 1 tablespoon of chili powder

Directions

- Firstly, set your Instant Pot to Sauté.
- Then, heat 2 tablespoons of olive oil.

- Add onion together with the garlic and fresh poblano, let sauté for 3 minutes until fragrant.
- Add canned chilies together with the canned beans and <u>jackfruit</u> .
- Add the <u>veggie broth</u> .
- Add all the spice along with <u>sugar</u> and <u>salt</u> .
- Stir and set <u>Instant pot</u> to a high heat for 10 minutes.
- Naturally release the pressure.
- Stir in corn with chopped kale and cover for 5 minutes on warm setting.
- Taste, and adjust the seasoning.
- Serve in bowls with diced <u>avocado</u> , cilantro, radishes.
- Serve and enjoy.

Moroccan red lentil quinoa soup

Ingredients

- 2 tablespoons of <u>olive oil</u>
- 1 teaspoon of <u>maple syrup</u>
- 1 teaspoon of dried thyme
- 1 teaspoon of <u>coriander</u>
- 1 onion, diced
- 3/4 cup of <u>red lentils</u>
- 6 garlic cloves, rough chopped
- 3 carrots, diced
- 1 red bell pepper, diced
- 1 teaspoon of <u>cinnamon</u>
- ¼ cup of quinoa
- 1 poblano pepper, diced
- 1 14-ounce can of diced tomatoes
- 4 cups <u>veggie broth</u>
- 1 ½ teaspoon of <u>salt</u>
- 2 teaspoons of <u>cumin</u>
- 1 teaspoon of chili powder
- ½ teaspoon of turmeric

Directions

- **Set** Instant Pot **to sauté function.**
- Heat olive oil.
- Then, sauté the onion and garlic for 4 minutes, stirring until fragrant.
- Add the carrots together with bell pepper, stir 2 minutes.
- Add the diced tomatoes and broth.
- Stir in the salt together with the cumin, chili powder, cinnamon, mable syrup, coriander, turmeric, and thyme .
- Stir in the split red lentils with the quinoa.
- Set instant pot to high pressure for 5 minutes.
- Manually release the pressure.
- Taste, and adjust the seasoning.
- Serve and enjoy with fresh radishes and herbs.

Potato wedges

Ingredients

- Olive oil
- Sea salt
- 600g of baking potatoes
- Freshly ground black pepper

Directions

- Firstly, preheat your oven ready to 400°F.
- Put a large pan of salted water to boil.
- Add the potato wedges to the pan of boiling water let boil for 8 minutes.
- Drain any excess water in a colander, let steam dry for briefly.
- Transfer to a roasting tray.
- Add olive oil together with a pinch of salt and pepper.
- Toss to coat the wedges with oil, spread out in one layer.
- Let cook in the hot oven for 30 minutes or until golden and cooked through.
- Serve and enjoy with chicken or a dip.

Brothy tortellini soup with spinach, white beans, and basil

Ingredients

- 1 can of white beans
- 2 tablespoons of <u>olive oil</u>
- 8 ounces of chopped baby spinach
- 1 onion, diced
- 6 garlic cloves, rough chopped
- 1 teaspoon of <u>salt</u>
- 1 cup of fresh basil, chopped
- ½ teaspoon of pepper
- 1 cup of celery, diced
- 10 ounces of fresh tortellini
- 8 cups of veggie
- Squeeze of lemon
- 1 teaspoon of dry Italian herbs

Directions

- Begin by heating olive oil in a large heavy bottom pot over medium-high heat.
- Add the onion to sauté for 4 minutes, stirring.

- Add the celery with garlic, lower heat to medium, let sauté for 6 minutes until celery is tender.
- Add the broth, then raise the heat to high, bring to a boil.
- Season with <u>salt</u> and Italian seasoning.
- Add the fresh tortellini when boiling, let simmer for 5 minutes or until cooked.
- Add the white beans and simmer briefly until heated through.
- Add the chopped fresh spinach together with the basil, after turning off the heat.
- Stir, and add a little squeeze of lemon.
- Taste, and adjust the seasoning.
- Serve and enjoy with a drizzle of <u>olive oil</u> , <u>pecorino</u> cheese and a light sprinkle of chili flakes.

Vegan ramen with shiitake broth

Ingredients

- 2 tablespoons of white <u>miso</u> paste
- 1 large onion-diced
- Pepper to taste
- 2 smashed garlic cloves
- Sriracha to taste
- 2 tablespoon of <u>olive oil</u>
- 8 ounces of <u>Ramen Noodles</u>
- 4 cups of <u>veggie stock</u>
- 8 ounces of cubed crispy tofu
- 4 cups of water
- ½ cup of <u>dried Shiitake</u> Mushrooms
- 1 sheet <u>Kombu</u> seaweed
- 1/8 cup of <u>mirin</u>

Directions

- **Sauté onion o** ver medium-high heat in 1 tablespoon olive oil until tender about 3 minutes.

- Turn heat to medium, add the smashed garlic cloves, let the onions cook until deeply golden brown.
- Add the veggie stock with water, dried shiitakes, a sheet of kombu , and mirin . Let Simmer for 30 minutes uncovered.
- R *emove the* Kombu .
- Then, add the miso with pepper to taste.
- In a pot of boiling water, cook the ramen noodles according to directions. Drain.
- Toss with sesame oil to keep separated.
- **Sauté the spinach and** mushrooms in olive oil until tender.
- Seasoning with salt and pepper.
- Fill bowls with cooked noodles, crispy tofu , and any other veggies.
- Pour the flavorful Shiitake broth over top.
- Serve and enjoy garnished with srirachi.

Cornbread casserole

Ingredients

- 2 large eggs
- 2 tablespoons of olive oil
- 1 cup of sour cream
- 1 onion, diced
- ¼ cup of melted butter
- 1 red bell pepper, diced
- 2 teaspoons of baking powder
- 4 cups of corn
- 1 ½ cups of grated cheese cheddar
- 4-ounce can of diced green chilies
- 1 teaspoon of cumin
- 1 teaspoon of coriander
- Salt
- 2 tablespoons chopped cilantro
- ½ cup of cornmeal
- 1 teaspoon of smoked paprika
- ½ cup of all-purpose flour
- 2 teaspoon of sugar

Directions

- In a large skillet, over medium heat, sauté onion in <u>olive oil</u> until fragrant in 4 minutes.
- Add the bell pepper, let cook for 4 minutes.
- Add the fresh corn and let sauté for 4 minutes.
- Stir in fresh cilantro.
- In a large bowl, combine cornmeal together with the salt, flour, baking powder, and sugar, whisk.
- In a separate medium bowl, whisk eggs with the sour cream. Then, gently whisk in the melted butter.
- Add the sautéed corn/pepper mixture to the dry ingredients with the egg mixture, stir to combine.
- Add 3/4 cup of grated cheese.
- Pour the batter into the greased baking dish.
- Topping with the remaining 3/4 cup of cheese.
- Bake for 35 minutes uncovered.
- Serve and enjoy warm sprinkled with cilantro.

Thai green curry

Ingredients

- Lime wedges for garnish
- ½ cup of <u>homemade green curry paste</u>
- 1 Japanese eggplant
- 1 teaspoon of <u>sugar</u>
- 2 tablespoons of olive <u>oil</u>
- 8 kefir lime leaves
- 1 cup of chicken broth
- ¼ cup of fresh Thai basil leaves, torn
- 1 can of <u>coconut milk</u>
- 8 ounces' pound of extra-firm tofu, cubed
- ½ teaspoon of <u>salt</u>
- 2 teaspoons of <u>fish sauce</u>
- 1 red bell pepper, sliced
- Lime juice to taste

Directions

- Begin by heating olive oil in a heavy bottom pot over medium-high heat.
- Stir-fry the homemade green curry paste for 3 minutes.

- Add the stock, then Stir in one can of full coconut milk .

- Add salt , sugar , and fish sauce

- Add the tofu together with the veggies and kefir lime leaves.

- Bring to a gentle simmer, uncovered until eggplant softens.

- Add a squeeze of lime and taste, and adjust accordingly.

- Add the fresh basil leaves and serve with lime wedges over rice.

- Enjoy.

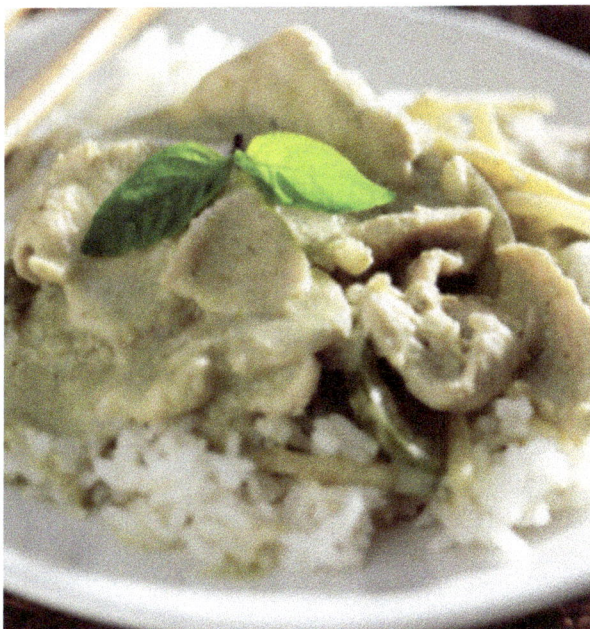

Kimchi burritos

Ingredients

- 1 cup of shredded cheese
- ½ cup of <u>kimchi</u> , chopped
- 2 tablespoon of <u>olive oil</u>
- 2 scallions, chopped
- 1 onion, diced
- Cilantro, hot sauce
- Salt to taste
- 1 red bell pepper, diced
- 1 cup of rice
- 1 can of black beans, rinsed, strained

Directions

- In a large skillet, heat oil over medium heat.
- Then, sauté onion with bell pepper for 5 minutes or until tender.
- Add rice together with <u>kimchi</u> and black beans, stir to combine.
- Season with <u>salt</u> and scallions.
- Taste, and adjust spices accordingly.

- Add cheese to the pan, gently melt, stirring for until melty and stringy.
- Divide filling into the center of the warm tortillas.
- Top with <u>hot sauce</u> and or cilantro and wrap into a burrito.
- Serve and enjoy immediately.

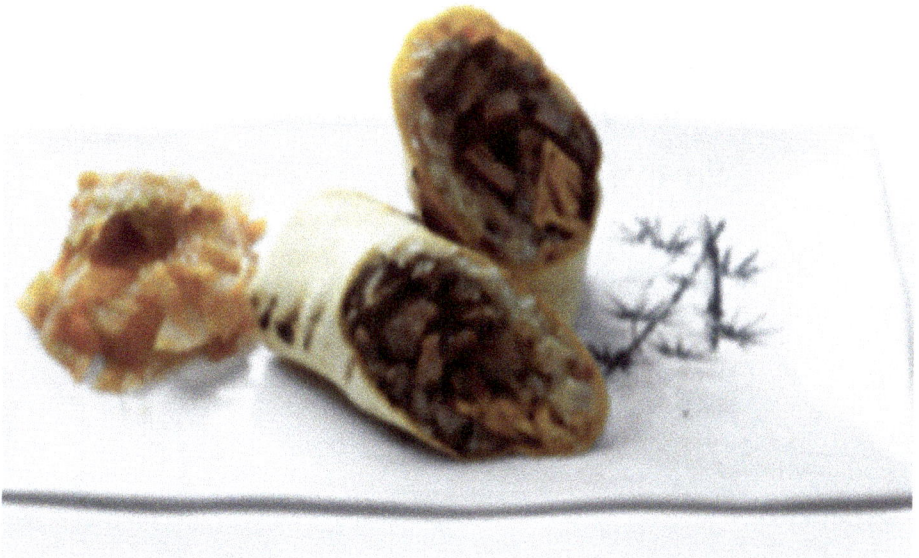

Singapore style fried rice

This specific Mediterranean Sea diet recipe has many variations with a perfect seasoning and fluffiness, if can be blended with various vegetables of your liking.

Ingredients

- 1 teaspoon of chili jam
- 4 fresh or frozen raw peeled prawns
- 150g of brown
- 1 teaspoon of mixed seeds
- 320g of crunchy veggies
- 1 tablespoon of low-salt soy sauce
- 1 teaspoon of tikka paste
- 1 rasher of smoked streaky bacon
- 1 clove of garlic
- 2cm of piece of ginger
- 1 large free-range egg
- Olive oil
- 1 chipolata

Directions

- Start by cooking the rice according as per packet Directions.

- Drain any excess water let cool.
- Put a large non-stick frying pan on a medium-high heat.
- Place 1 teaspoon of olive oil into the hot pan.
- Pour in the egg, swirl around the pan.
- Cook through, remove and roll up and slice.
- Put ½ a tablespoon of olive oil into the hot pan.
- Stir-fry the bacon with sausages until golden.
- Add the prawns with garlic and ginger.
- Stir in the curry paste to coated everything.
- Add the vegetables, begin with hard to cook veggies. Keep stirring.
- Place in the cool rice and stir-fry until the veggies are just cooked.
- Add the soy, toss in the egg ribbons.
- Divide between plates, sprinkle over the seeds.
- Season and adjust accordingly.
- Serve and enjoy with a drizzle of chili jam.

Purple cauliflower salad

Ingredients

- 2 tablespoons of <u>red wine vinegar</u>
- ½ cup of Italian parsley, chopped
- 1 head cauliflower
- ½ teaspoon of pepper
- 2 cloves garlic, minced
- Salt
- zest of one lemon
- 2 cups of cooked grain- <u>black rice</u>
- 2 scallions, sliced
- ½ cup of sliced Kalamata olives
- 2 tablespoons of <u>capers</u>
- <u>olive oil</u>

<u>Directions</u>

- Preheat your oven to 425°F.
- Set grains to cook on the stove.
- Remove and let cool.
- Cut cauliflower into bite-sized florets.
- Then, slightly toss in <u>olive oil</u> , <u>salt</u> and lemon zest.

- Spread out on a <u>parchment</u> -lined baking sheet.
- Let roast for 25 minutes, turning halfway through. Let cool.
- In a bowl, whisk olive oil, red wine vinegar, garlic, salt, and pepper.
- Layer salad ingredients in a shallow bowl starting with the grain.
- Serve and enjoy.

Grilled cabbage with andouille sausage

Ingredients

- 1 tablespoon of <u>olive oil</u>
- 1 tablespoon of fresh chives
- 2 tablespoons of <u>whole grain mustard</u>
- 1 ½ tablespoons of <u>honey</u>
- 1 large purple cabbage
- <u>Olive oil</u> for brushing
- Salt and pepper
- 6 andouille sausages
- ¼ teaspoon of <u>salt</u>
- ¼ teaspoon of pepper
- 2 tablespoons of <u>apple cider vinegar</u>

Directions

- Preheat your <u>grill</u> on high heat.
- Grease the <u>grill</u> well.
- Brush each side of cabbage with <u>olive oil</u> .
- Season with <u>salt</u> and pepper.
- lower <u>grill</u> to medium heat, then add sausages and thinly sliced cabbage.
- <u>Grill</u> the cabbage for 8 minutes on both sides.

- <u>Grill</u> the sausages until seared.
- Place cabbage steaks down on a large platter.
- Spoon half of the dressing over top.
- Slice the sausages in half and steep diagonal and scatter over cabbage.
- Serve and enjoy garnished with chopped chives.

Superfood walnut pesto noodles

Ingredients

- ¼ cup of sliced radishes
- 1 cup of walnuts
- ¼ cup of walnuts
- 2 tablespoons of <u>sesame oil</u>
- 4 ounces of dry <u>soba noodles</u>
- 1 cup of power greens
- Squeeze of lemon to taste
- 2 tablespoons of white <u>miso</u>
- <u>Olive oil</u> and lemon for drizzling
- 2 garlic cloves, start with one
- ¼ cup water
- 4 cups of baby superfood greens
- ½ cup of shredded cabbage
- Edamame, sunflower sprouts, <u>avocado</u>, snow peas

Directions

- Cook soba noodles according to the package ins

- Place walnuts together with the <u>miso</u> , olive oil, garlic, and water into a food processor, blend repeatedly.
- Then, add the power greens and pulse.
- Taste and adjust the taste and consistence.
- Toss the noodles with walnut pesto.
- Place noodles in a bento box with a handful of greens, shredded cabbage, walnuts, and radishes.
- Drizzle vegetables with a little <u>olive oil</u> , lemon, and <u>salt</u> .
- Serve and enjoy.

Carrots soup with chermoula

Ingredients

- ½ a large onion
- 1 tablespoon of lemon juice
- 1 ½ teaspoon of <u>Cumin seeds</u>
- ¼ teaspoon of <u>salt</u>
- 4 garlic cloves, smashed
- 4 cups chicken stock
- 2 bay leaves
- Zest from ½ lemon
- 1 teaspoon of <u>kosher salt</u>
- ¼ teaspoon of <u>white pepper</u>
- ¼ teaspoon of chili flakes
- 2 teaspoons of <u>honey</u>
- ¼ cup of yogurt
- 1 teaspoon of <u>cumin seeds</u> , toasted
- 1 lbs. carrots, cut into disks
- 1 teaspoon of fresh thyme
- 1 teaspoon coriander seeds, toasted
- 1 cup of cilantro
- ½ cup of Italian parsley

- 1 teaspoon of fresh ginger
- 2 garlic cloves
- Olive oil

Directions

- Sauté onion together with the <u>cumin seeds</u> and smashed garlic in olive oil over medium high heat until golden, stirring often.
- Add carrots with chicken stock, bay leaves, <u>salt</u> , <u>white pepper</u> .
- Bring to a vigorous simmer, lower, simmer covered for 20 minutes over low heat.
- Then, toast the spices in a dry skillet over medium heat until fragrant.
- Combine all ingredients in a <u>food processor</u> , blend to form paste. Keep aside for later.
- Blend the soup using an immersion blender or in small batches.
- Place back in the pot, stir in sour cream and <u>maple syrup</u> .
- Taste, and adjust seasoning.
- Divide among bowls, then add a spoonful of chermoula, swirl in a circle.

- Serve and enjoy.

Lemony corona beans with olive and garlic

Ingredients

- Salt and pepper to taste
- 2 teaspoons of kosher salt
- ¼ cup of fresh parsley leaves
- 2 bay leaves
- 3 celery sticks, cut into pieces
- Aleppo chili flakes
- 1 onion, quartered
- zest of one lemon
- 1 lb. dry Royal Corona Beans
- 4 garlic cloves, smashed
- A few fresh sage leaves
- 3 tablespoons of olive oil

Directions

- Place soaked beans in a large Dutch oven with water enough to cover them.
- Add salt together with the celery, garlic, onion, bay leaves, and herbs.

- Bring to a boil, lower heat, let simmer covered until tender n about 2 hours.
- Drain, reserve some liquid without the aromatics for later.
- Place in a <u>serving dish</u> .
- Then, add back 1 cup of the reserved warm cooking liquid with <u>olive oil</u> , lemon zest, fresh Italian parsley, and <u>salt</u> and pepper.
- Serve and enjoy.

Szechuan tofu and vegetables

Ingredients

- 1 cup of asparagus, snap peas
- 12 ounces of tofu, patted dry, cubed
- ¼ cup of Szechuan Sauce
- 1 cup of shredded carrots
- 2 tablespoons of peanut oil
- generous pinch of salt and pepper
- ½ red bell pepper, thinly sliced
- ½ cup of thinly sliced onion
- Scallions of sesame seeds
- 4 ounces of sliced mushrooms
- 2 cups of shredded cabbage

Directions

- Heat olive oil in a skillet over medium heat.
- Season peanut oil together with salt and pepper.
- Then, swirl the seasoned peanut oil to spread out uniformly.
- Add tofu and sear on at least two sides, until crispy and golden.

- In the same pan, add onion and mushrooms.
- Sauté over medium-high heat, stirring constantly, until tender.
- Add the remaining vegetables with dried red chilies
- Lower heat to medium, sauté, while tossing and stirring for 5 minutes.
- Add the Szechuan Sauce , gradually.
- Let cook for 2 minutes, until thickened a bit.
- Toss in the crispy tofu towards the end.
- Divide among bowls.
- Sprinkle with sesame seeds and scallions.
- Serve and enjoy with noodles or over rice.

Kyoto roasted sweet potatoes with miso, ginger, and scallions

Ingredients

- Salt to taste
- 3 yams sliced in half
- 2 teaspoons of ginger finely minced
- 3 Scallions, sliced
- Olive oil for brushing
- 1 tablespoon of <u>miso</u>
- ¼ cup of <u>olive oil</u>
- 1 large shallot, finely diced

Directions

- Preheat your oven ready to 425°F.
- Place cut sweet potatoes on a <u>parchment</u> -lined <u>sheet pan</u>
- Brush with <u>olive oil</u> .
- Let roast for 40 minutes until fork tender.
- Heat the olive oil over medium low heat.
- Then, add the shallot to sauté until golden, stirring often.

- Add the ginger, continue to cook for 3 more minutes.
- Add and mash the <u>miso</u> with a fork into the mixture. Turn off the heat.
- After the sweet potatoes are caramelized, remove and place on a platter flesh side up.
- Reheat the miso, pierce the flesh in a few spots, spoon a tablespoon of the sauce over each one with the flavor.
- Sprinkle with a little <u>finishing salt</u> and scallions.
- Serve and enjoy.